DORSAF ALOUI
MERIAM BOUCHEKOUA
SONIA TRABELSI

What about imported bilharziasis in Tunisia?

DORSAF ALOUI
MERIAM BOUCHEKOUA
SONIA TRABELSI

What about imported bilharziasis in Tunisia?

Bilharziasis among non-permanent resident students in Tunisia: epidemiological and parasitological profile

ScienciaScripts

Imprint

Cover image: www.ingimage.com

This book is a translation from the original published under ISBN 978-613-8-46670-3.

Publisher:
Sciencia Scripts
is a trademark of
Dodo Books Indian Ocean Ltd. and OmniScriptum S.R.L publishing group

120 High Road, East Finchley, London, N2 9ED, United Kingdom
Str. Armeneasca 28/1, office 1, Chisinau MD-2012, Republic of Moldova, Europe
Printed at: see last page
ISBN: 978-620-8-26668-4

TABLE OF CONTENTS

INTRODUCTION

Bilharziasis or shistosomiasis is the world's second most common parasitic disease after malaria. Despite control efforts in many tropical and subtropical countries, the World Health Organisation (WHO) estimated that in 2021 at least 251.4 million people needed preventive treatment against schistosomiasis, while 75.3 million people needed treatment [1].

Schistosoma (S.), the causative agent, is a transcutaneously transmitted parasite of visceral venous plexuses, with freshwater molluscs as intermediate hosts. The migration and embolisation of bilharzia eggs in the circulatory system are responsible for hepatosplenic and urogenital complications, which can be fatal. Mortality is estimated at 54 million deaths every year [1].

In Tunisia, thanks to the implementation of national eradication programmes, indigenous transmission of urinary bilharziasis, the only form that existed, was halted in 1984. However, we are currently witnessing the emergence of a new epidemiological profile represented by imported cases, which are constantly on the increase, posing a potential risk of their reintroduction into Tunisia [2].

As part of the maintenance phase of the national programme to eradicate bilharziasis and malaria and to monitor emerging and re-emerging intestinal and urinary parasitoses in our country, parasitological surveillance of students who are not permanent residents of Tunisia (ENRPT) is of particular interest. When they enrol at university, they undergo a systematic medical examination at the School and University Medical Centre and a parasitological examination of stools (EPS) and urine (EPU). In this work, we set out to draw up an epidemiological, clinical and parasitological profile of bilharziasis diagnosed in ENRPTs.

MATERIALS AND METHODS

1.TYPE OF STUDY

This was a cross-sectional, descriptive study carried out in the Parasitology-Mycology laboratory at Charles Nicolle Hospital in Tunis over a period of fifteen academic years, from 2008-2009 to 2022-2023. It focused on ENRPTs pursuing their university studies in various state and private institutions in the Tunis region.

2.STUDY POPULATION

2.1. Inclusion criteria

All ENRPT sent to the Parasitology-Mycology laboratory at the Charles Nicolle Hospital in Tunis by the Department of School and University Medicine as part of the national surveillance programme for emerging and re-emerging intestinal and urinary parasitoses.

2.2. Non inclusion criteria

Tunisians and foreigners referred to the laboratory on suspicion of bilharziasis.

3.DATA COLLECTION METHOD

All the data required for the study were collected using a clinical-epidemiological information sheet.

4.PARASITOLOGICAL EXAMINATION OF STOOLS

4.1. Conditions for direct debit

Sampling conditions were required before any PHE.

• The sample should be taken three to four days after the patient has stopped taking certain drugs that may interfere with its interpretation, such as paraffin oil and intestinal dressings.

• Avoid fruit and vegetables for two days before sampling (prefer a low-residue diet).

• Collect the faeces in a clean, hermetically sealed jar.

• Forward stools immediately (<1 hour) (do not freeze or store in a cool place).

• Avoid urine contamination

4.2. Macroscopic examination of stools

Macroscopic examination of the stools was as follows:

- Assess stool colour and consistency.

- Note the presence of blood or mucus or macroscopic elements such as tapeworm rings or adult pinworms, indicating polyparasitism.

4.3. Microscopic examination of stools

4.3.1. Examination direct

Direct examination reveals helminth eggs, including schistosomes (the 5 species of Schistosoma sp), helminth larvae and the vegetative and cystic forms of protozoa that may be associated with them. It was carried out by diluting a dab of stool in a drop of physiological water on a slide. Microscopic observation was carried out using a x10 objective and then a x40 objective.

4.3.2. Concentration technique

The concentration technique used in the laboratory was the simplified Ritchie technique, which is a physico-chemical method. It was carried out systematically, thereby increasing the sensitivity of the search for helminth eggs and protozoan cysts.

This technique consisted of :

➢ Carefully crush a stool mass in a volume of 10% isotonic formalin solution.

➢ Filter the resulting mixture through a sieve into a 30 ml conical tube.

➢ Centrifuge at 1500 rpm for 2 minutes.

➢ Remove the supernatant.

➢ Resuspend in 7 mL of 10% formalin and add 3 mL of ethyl acetate.

➢ Close the tube and shake vigorously to emulsify the mixture.

➢ Centrifuge at 1500 rpm for two minutes.

➢ Remove the supernatant and examine the pellet at x10 and then x40 magnification.

5. PARASITOLOGICAL EXAMINATION OF URINE

5.1.Conditions for direct debit

Urine was collected in the morning in a clean container. To increase the sensitivity of this examination, the student was asked to perform a suprapubic massage or physical effort (hopping, climbing stairs, walking, etc.) to remove the eggs from the bladder wall.

5.2.Macroscopic examination of urine

Macroscopic examination of the urine revealed the appearance of the urine (clear, cloudy) and the presence or absence of haematuria.

5.3.Microscopic examination of urine

Direct examination was used to detect S. haematobium eggs. The procedure was as follows:

• Centrifuge the urine at 3000 rpm for five minutes.

• Remove the supernatant.

• Examine the pellet at ×10 and then ×40.

6.DECLARATION OF POSITIVE CASES

All parasitic patients were declared by filling in the notification form for notifiable transmissible diseases on the register provided by the basic healthcare department. All these parasitic patients were subsequently referred by the School and University Medical Department to the Infectious Diseases Department for treatment and follow-up.

7.STATISTICAL ANALYSIS METHODS

The data were entered and analysed using IBM SPSS Statistics software version 26.0. Simple frequencies and relative frequencies (percentages) were used to calculate the qualitative variables. Means and medians were determined for quantitative variables.

8.BIBLIOGRAPHIC RESEARCH METHODS

Bibliographic research was carried out by consulting the main scientific sources on the Internet. The main scientific search enginesused were Pubmed (http://www.ncbi.nlm.nih.gov/pubmed) and Science direct (http://www.sciencedirect.com). .

The keywords used were: urogenital bilharziasis, intestinal bilharziasis, non-permanent resident students in Tunisia and their equivalents in English. The bibliography was organised using Zotero version 6.0 software.

9.ETHICAL CONSIDERATIONS AND CONFLICTS OF INTEREST

- This study was carried out for academic, not-for-profit purposes.

- Anonymity and medical confidentiality were respected.

- There was no conflict of interest.

RESULTS

1. OVERALL RESULTS

During the study period, which spanned 15 academic years (2008 - 2023), 6051 NPRTs were sent to the laboratory.

Schistosomiasis was diagnosed in 91 students, a frequency of 1.5%, distributed as follows:

- Intestinal schistosomiasis was found in 77 students (83%)
- Urogenital shistosomiasis was diagnosed in 15 students (16.4%)
- One student had a combination of both clinical forms (Figure 1).

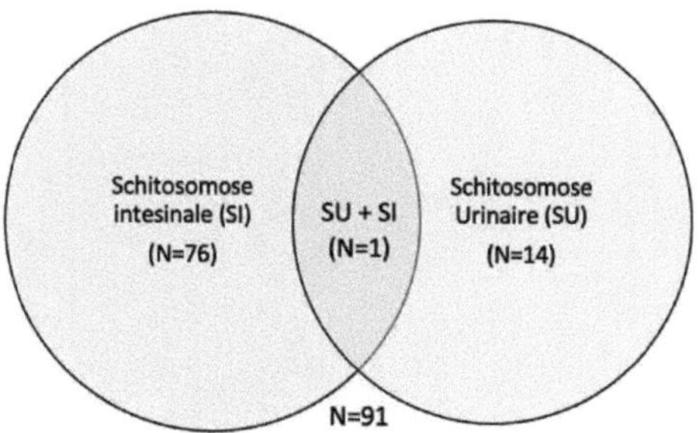

Figure 1: Breakdown of schistosomiasis cases

1.1. Breakdown of patients by age

The mean age of patients with parasites was 24.4 ± 4.14 years, with extremes ranging from 17 to 38 years. The 20-30 age group accounted for 81% of the parasitized population (Figure 2).

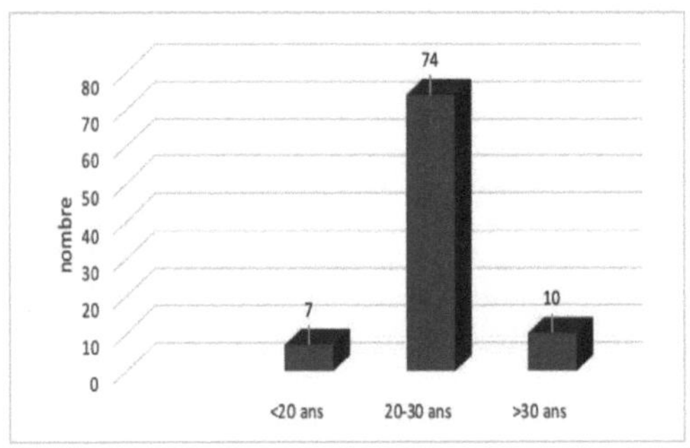

Figure 2: Age distribution of patients

1.2. Breakdown of patients by gender

A clear male predominance was found in our patients: 70 men (77%) for 21 women, i.e. a M/F sex ratio of 3.33.

1.3. Breakdown of patients by geographical origin

Geographical origin was specified for 89 students. All were from sub-Saharan Africa. Students from the Ivory Coast and Congo were the most affected, with 23 and 21 cases respectively, followed by those from Guinea (16 cases) and Cameroon (8 cases) (Table I).

Table I: Distribution of parasitized ENRPT according to geographical origin

Geographical origin	Workforce	%
Ivory Coast	23	26
Democratic Republic of Congo (DRC)	21	23
Guinea	16	18
Cameroon	8	9
Mali	3	4
Burkina Faso	3	4
Mauritania	3	4
Gabon	2	2
Zambia	2	2
Chad	2	2
Nigeria	2	2
Central African Republic	1	1
Madagascar	1	1
Gambia	1	1
Senegal	1	1
Total	89	100

1.4. Number of cases by year

The trend in cases over the years showed a very heterogeneous distribution, with a peak in the 2017-2018 academic year and no cases in the 2010-2011 and 2022-2023 academic years (Figure 3).

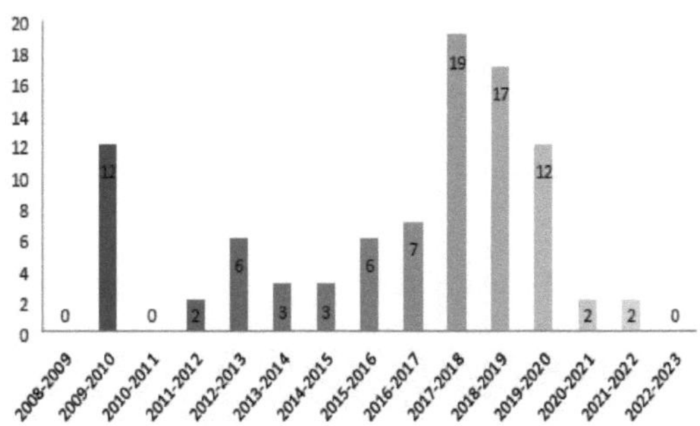

Figure 3: Annual breakdown of diagnosed cases

2. SCHISTOSOMIASIS INTESTINAL

Isolated intestinal schistosomiasis was noted in 83% of cases (N =76), i.e. in 1.3% of all students referred to the laboratory during the study period. All cases involved S. mansoni, which was the only species isolated from the faeces.

2.1.Epidemiological profile of patients

2.1.1. Age

The mean age of NERPT with intestinal schistosomiasis was 24.8 ± 4.3 years, with extremes ranging from 17 to 38 years.

2.1.2. Type

Intestinal schistosomiasis was most frequently found in men, in 76% of cases (N=59), with a sex ratio of 3.47.

2.1.3.Geographical origin

The majority of NEPTs with intestinal schistosomiasis were from Côte d'Ivoire (26%, N=20) and Congo (25%, N=19) (Figure 4).

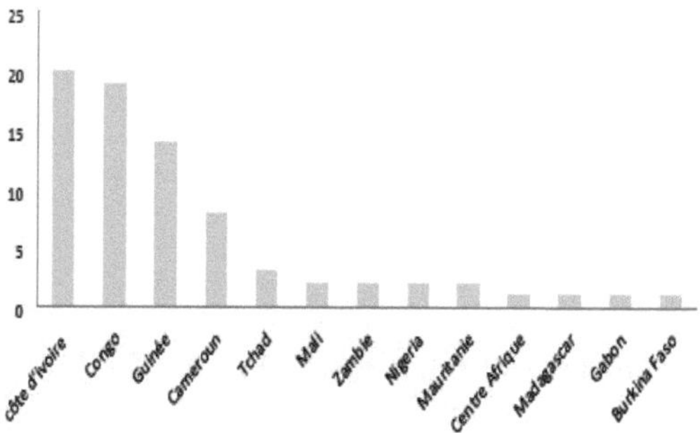

Figure 4: Distribution of intestinal schistosomiasis cases according to geographical origin

2.2.Clinical profile

2.2.1. History of schistosomiasis

When questioned, only one student reported a treated episode of intestinal schistosomiasis caused by S. mansoni.

2.2.2. Clinical symptoms

Only 4 of the 76 students with parasites mentioned the presence of clinical signs such as diarrhoea, fever or isolated abdominal pain.

2.3. Parasitological profile

The diagnosis of this infection was made by the detection of S. mansoni eggs in all cases, thanks to parasitological examination of the faeces. Apart from the student who had a combination of both clinical forms of bilharziasis, whose results will be detailed later, polyparasitism (a combination of S. mansoni and other intestinal parasites) was noted in 47 patients (62%), while only 29 had S. mansoni alone. An association of 3 or more parasites was noted in 40% of cases (N= 19) (Table II).

Table II: Distribution of polyparasitism according to geographical origin in cases of intestinal shistosomiasis

Origin geographical	Number of patients infested	S. mansoni alone	Polyparasitism
Ivory Coast	20	5	15
RDC	19	7	12
Guinea	14	8	6
Cameroon	8	3	5
Chad	3	1	2
Mali	2	0	2
Zambia	2	1	1
Nigeria	2	1	1
Mauritania	2	1	1
Africa Centre	1	1	0
Madagascar	1	0	1
Gabon	1	1	0
Burkina Faso	1	0	1
Total	76	29 (38%)	47 (62%)

A total of 77 digestive parasites associated with S. mansoni were isolated from these 47 ENRPT. The associations were essentially with protozoa, with a frequency of 87% (67/77), the majority of which were non-pathogenic, with Endolimax nanus in first place (26 cases), followed by Entamoeba coli (18 cases). For pathogenic protozoa, only one case of association was noted with Entamoeba histolytica. An association with helminths, parasites that are pathogenic for humans, was found in 10 cases (Table III).

Table III: Typology of parasites associated with S. mansoni

Protozoa		Helminths	
Species	Workforce	Species	Workforce
Endolimax nanus	26	Hookworm	4
Entamoeba coli	18	Anguillule	3
Entamoeba hartmanni	7	Trichuris trichura	1
Blastocystissp	11	Ascaris	2
Chilomastix mesnili	1		
Cystoisospora belli	1		
Entamoeba histolytica	1		
Iodamoeba butschli	2		
Total	67	Total	10

3. UROGENITAL SCHISTOSOMIASIS

Isolated urogenital shistosomiasis was diagnosed in 14 ERNPT (15.3% of schistosomes), i.e. in 0.2% of the students referred to the laboratory during the study period.

3.1.Epidemiological profile of patients

3.1.1. Age

The average age of the students in whom urogenital schistosomiasis was identified was 23.4±2.25 years, with extremes ranging from 18 to 27 years.

3.1.2. Type

These ENRPTs (11) were predominantly male, with a sex ratio of 3.6.

3.1.3. Geographical origin

The majority of NEPTs were from sub-Saharan Africa (Figure 5).

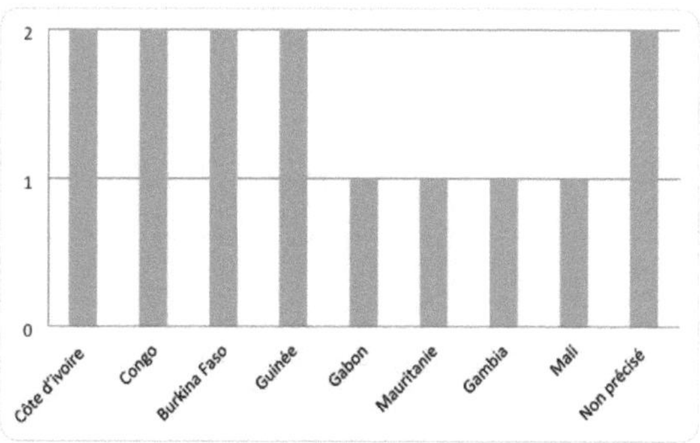

Figure 5: Distribution of urogenital shistosomiasis cases according to geographical origin

3.2.Clinical profile

3.2.1. History of urogenital schistosomiasis

During questioning, no history of urogenital schistosomiasis was reported in any of the ERNPT patients.

3.2.2. Clinical symptoms

N o suggestive symptomatology (haematuria, etc.) was found in NNPT with urinary schistosomiasis.

3.3.Parasitological profile

Urogenital shistosomiasis was diagnosed by the detection of eggs of S. haematobium (the only species responsible for this clinical form). Apart from the student who had a combination of the two clinical forms of bilharziasis, whose results will be detailed later, polyparasitism (a combination of S. haematobium and other intestinal parasites) was noted in 8 patients (Table IV).Of the thirteen (13) associated parasites, 9 were protozoa, all of which were non-pathogenic. Helminths were found in 4 patients.

Table IV: Distribution of polyparasitism according to geographical origin in cases of urogenital schistosomiasis

Origin geographical	Number of infested patients	Parasitism (S.hematobium alone)	Polyparasitism
Congo	2	1	1
Ivory Coast	2	1	1
Guinea	2	1	1
Not specified	2	1	1
Gabon	1	0	1
Gambia	1	0	1
Mauritania	1	0	1
Mali	1	0	1
Burkina Faso	2	2	0
Total	14	6	8

4.ASSOCIATION OF THE TWO CLINICAL FORMS OF SCHISTOSOMIASIS :

A combination of urogenital and intestinal schistosomiasis was found in only one student.

4.1.Epidemiological profile of the patient

She was a student, aged 30. She was originally from Côte d'Ivoire.

4.2.Clinical Profile

During questioning, no history of schistosomiasis was reported in this patient. No clinical signs (digestive and/or urinary) were found in her.

4.3. Parasitological profile

This association was diagnosed by the detection of S. haematobium and S. mansoni eggs in the student's urine and faeces respectively. No other associated parasites were isolated from the patient.

DISCUSSION

Bilharzia is a parasite that has been eliminated in Tunisia since 1984. Currently, there are only imported cases. As part of the programme to control emerging and re-emerging intestinal and urinary parasites, screening for NPPTs is essential to prevent the reintroduction of this parasite. It consists of carrying out an EPS and EPU on all foreign students, who are referred to the parasitology laboratories in Tunis, prior to their enrolment in Tunisian institutions. Against this backdrop, this study looks at the epidemiological and parasitological characteristics of intestinal and urogenital bilharziasis found in ERNPT. A retrospective descriptive study was conducted over a period of fifteen academic years (from 2008/2009 to 2022/2023) in the Parasitology-Mycology laboratory at Charles Nicolle Hospital in Tunis. It focused on 91 students with schistosomiasis (intestinal, urogenital or associated) out of a total of 6051 students screened during the same period, representing a frequency of 1.5%. Intestinal schistosomiasis was diagnosed in 76 ENRPT (83% of cases), whereas urogenital schistosomiasis was less common and was found in only 14 students. A combination of the two clinical forms of schistosomiasis was isolated in only one case. Positive cases were reported to the

Basic Healthcare Department to ensure that patients received appropriate treatment. The average age of the ENRPT parasitized was 24±4.14 years, with a clear male predominance (77%). They all originated from sub-Saharan Africa. Our study of schistosomes is the most recent in Tunisia. It has made it possible to update the epidemiological profile and the evolution of the prevalence of these emerging infections in the population studied, thanks to the large number of people studied. Our results reflect the persistence of the risk of reintroduction of these parasites in our country and the usefulness of maintaining systematic screening in this student population.However, like any study, it has its limitations, mainly due to the retrospective collection of data and its monocentric nature. Similarly, despite the mandatory reporting of positive cases to the Basic Health Care Department (DSSB), no post-treatment follow-up or parasitological checks were carried out.

A multicentre study would have enabled better control and management of the risk of reintroduction of these parasites in Tunisia.

1. OVERALL RESULTS

During the study period, 91 cases of schistosomiasis were recorded among 6051 ENRPT referred to the laboratory, giving a frequency of 1.5%. According to a similar study conducted at La Rabta Hospital in Tunis between 1990 and 2012, the frequency of ENRPT with this parasitosis was 2.02% [1]. In a study carried out in the parasitology laboratory at the Institut Pasteur in Tunis on the same study population between 1998 and 2002, the frequency was only 0.9% [2].

The average age of the students affected was 24.4 years, with a clear male predominance.Our data are consistent with the literature. In a study carried out in Europe over a period of 14 years, an average age of 28 years was reported, with a 71% male predominance [3]. Regarding geographical origin, all parasitized students were from sub-Saharan Africa (Ivory Coast, DRC, Guinea). These results were similar to work carried out in 2018 and 2019 in Italy [4,5]. According to the latest figures, it is estimated that almost 90% of patients suffering from bilharzia originate from sub-Saharan Africa (Nigeria, Ivory Coast, DRC, etc.) and that 280,000 deaths secondary to this parasite are recorded there each year [6].

2. INTESTINAL SCHISTOSOMIASIS

Intestinal schistosomiasis was diagnosed in 1.3% of all students referred to the laboratory during the study period. All cases were due to S. mansoni, which was the only species implicated. According to the various Tunisian studies, this frequency varied from 0.03% to 3.43% (Table V).

Table V: Frequency of intestinal schistosomiasis among ENRPT in the various Tunisian studies

Authors	Study period	Frequency of schistosomiasis intestinal (%)
Chaker et al [7]	1984 - 1988	3,43
Siala et al [2]	1998 - 2002	0,03
Dridi et al [1]	1990 - 2012	1,26
Our study	2008 - 2023	1,3

This variability in detection rates for intestinal schistosomiasis may be explained by the fact that the figures may be underestimated. For reasons of cost and feasibility, screening for parasitosis in ENRPTs is limited to a single examination, whereas it is known that repeated examinations increase the sensitivity of investigations.This is related to the irregular and intermittent elimination of eggs and their rarity in samples, particularly when the subjects are pauci-parasitised and asymptomatic, as is the case for ENRPT [8-10]. In our study, S. mansoni eggs were only detected by the modified Ritchie concentration technique, whereas direct examination was negative in all cases. This could be explained by the low level of infestation in the parasitized students, most of whom were asymptomatic. Although the simplified Ritchie technique used in our study allows good stool concentration for the detection of schistosome eggs, there are more sensitive techniques such as the Kato technique. In an Italian study, it was concluded that it is indeed a question of is a highly sensitive technique for detecting helminth eggs and should be used in epidemiological surveys [11].

Sub-Saharan Africa was the origin of all students with intestinal schistosomiasis, mainly Côte d'Ivoire (26%, N=20) and Congo (25%, N=19). This distribution is consistent with that found in the literature [12,13].

Schistosomiasis is a major public health problem, particularly in sub-Saharan Africa. Nigeria, in West Africa, currently has the highest prevalence of schistosomiasis in the world.S. mansoni, the species responsible for American and African intestinal schistosomiasis, is found throughout Africa with the exception of the Maghreb [14]. It occurs throughout sub-Saharan Africa, with the exception of arid regions and the southern part of the continent. There are also pockets of transmission in the Nile delta in Egypt. However, mass treatment has significantly reduced its prevalence [6].

Despite the persistence of cases of imported S. mansoni in Tunisia, this parasite remains harmless under our skies due to the absence of molluscs, the intermediate host of this species, thus preventing the complete development of the intestinal bilharziosis cycle and its emergence.

In addition, 62% of our patients with intestinal schistosomiasis were polyparasitic. This clearly illustrates that these diseases are the result of exposure to faecal peril. Our data are consistent with the literature [15,16].

Although the protozoa identified are not pathogenic, their presence in faeces indicates poor hygiene. Given that the modes of transmission of digestive protozoa and helminths are equivalent, a person carrying a non-pathogenic parasite should be considered at risk because he or she may harbour other potentially pathogenic protozoa. Hookworm and anguillosis, transcutaneous parasitoses, have become rare in our country. They were identified in association with bilharziasis in our series. Their presence, which is not negligible, should encourage the continued use of specific techniques to detect these two parasites, such as the Baermann extraction technique and coproculture.

The clinical profile showed that only four students had digestive symptoms. In the course of intestinal bilharziasis, clinical signs evolve according to the evolutionary stages of the parasite, in three phases of unequal importance. Hepatosplenic involvement, which is frequent and late in cases of infestation by S. mansoni, is part of the final phase of visceral focalisation. It follows the phases of cercarial infestation and invasion, which are clinically inconsistent [17].

3. UROGENITAL SCHISTOSOMIASIS

Urogenital bilharziasis waś diagnosed in 14 ERNPT (15.3%of all schistosomiasis cases) or 0.2% of students referred to the laboratory during the study period. According to an earlier study carried out in our laboratory between 2005 and 2010, the frequency of urinary bilharziasis was higher (0.91%) [15], whereas it was only 0.1% in the study by Siala et al [4]. The rates were 29.3% and 10.5% respectively according to Buonfrate et al and Delcor et al [18,19].

The much lower frequencies observed in the Tunisian studies could be explained by the fact that the figures may be underestimated due to the low elimination of eggs in urine, which is intermittent over time. In order to increase the sensitivity of the parasitological examination of urine, it is recommended to collect urine between 10 a.m. and 2 p.m. (the time of day when egg concentration is at its highest) or the final 24 hours of urine. It is also advisable to collect urine after physical exertion, such as climbing stairs [20]. The multiplicity of urine samples would also increase the sensitivity of this test. Students do not always comply with all these conditions. As with intestinal schistosomiasis, ENRPT with urogenital schistosomiasis were predominantly male (N=11) with a mean age of 23.4±2.25 years. Several studies have found concordant results [21,22]. Schistosomiasis is transmitted to humans via furcocercariae (the infesting form of the parasite), which penetrate the skin after prolonged contact with freshwater. In such cases, men are more exposed because of fishing, rice-growing and swimming activities [20]. The countries of origin of ENRPT with urinary schistosomiasis were those of sub-Saharan Africa (Côte d'Ivoire, Burkina Faso, etc.), which is in line with the results of a recent Italian study [23].

S. haematobium is the causative agent of urogenital schistosomiasis. It is rife in Africa, mainly in sub-Saharan Africa (arid southern regions, southern Africa), the Nile Valley in Egypt and Sudan, the Maghreb and the Arabian Peninsula [14,24].It should be noted that a significant drop in the prevalence of urinary schistosoma (from 40-60% in 1935 to 1-10% in 2000) was observed in Egypt following the construction of the Aswan High Dam [25].

In North Africa, namely Tunisia and Morocco, bilharzia has been eliminated. However, it persists in Algeria and Libya according to the latest studies carried out in 2012 [26]. Since then, no updated data have been found. Since the beginning of the 20ème century, the south of Tunisia has been identified as an endemic area for S. haematobium schistosomiasis. The country has had three endemic foci in the regions of Gafsa, Kebili and Tozeur, with expansion northwards, affecting the Kairouan region in particular. In 1970, Tunisia implemented a national programme to eradicate urogenital bilharziasis, in collaboration with the WHO, using praziquantel to treat infected people, as well as molluscicides, such as bayluscide, to target molluscs, in particular Bulinus truncatus, an intermediate host for the parasite. And it was in 1984 that the last case of indigenous transmission was recorded in Tunisia, making the country the first in Africa to put a permanent end to transmission of the disease [27-29].

At present, the persistence of imported cases of urinary bilharziasis among individuals originating from endemic regions, combined with the high density of the bulin mollusc, an intermediate host of this parasitic disease, in the north of Tunisia (particularly in the regions of Tabarka, Kef and Cap Bon), represents a potential risk of resumption of indigenous transmission and re-emergence of this parasitosis in Tunisia. Consequently, it is justified to consider the systematic performance of parasitological examinations of urine for all persons coming from regions heavily affected by bilharziasis, in particular ENRPT, in order to prevent the re-emergence of this parasitosis [7].

It is essential to maintain a high level of vigilance, especially as autochthonous outbreaks of bilharziasis are beginning to emerge, as is the case in Corsica where 12 individuals were diagnosed with urinary bilharziasis after being exposed to a river in Corse-du-Sud and without having stayed in an endemic area for the disease [30]. Clinically, all patients were asymptomatic. In a study by Deniaud et al, 10 of 25 patients were found to have no urinary symptoms [31]. It is important to stress that clinical manifestations only occur in less than 10% of infected individuals, especially as they depend on factors linked to both the parasite and the host [32].

Polyparasitism was identified in 8 students with urogenital schistosomiasis, with evidence of a combination of urinary and intestinal schistosomiasis in one student. Several studies conducted in Senegal and in Italy showed an association of S. mansoni and S.

haematobium in 2% and 5.8% of cases respectively [4,33].

The presence of helminths in the PSE in addition to urinary schistosomiasis was noted in four students. The presence of these intestinal parasites highlights the importance of maintaining systematic coprological surveillance among ENRPTs, with the aim of preventing the introduction and spread of intestinal parasitosis in the country.

In addition to regular screening and compulsory reporting of bilharziasis, early and effective treatment is essential to avoid complications. The first-line treatment of choice for these parasites is Biltricide (Praziquantel ®), an antihelminthic which is not covered by the Tunisian hospital nomenclature and is only issued by the DSSB of the Ministry of Health. It is currently used in clinical practice, both for individual treatment and for mass treatment campaigns. However, forms of resistance to treatment are currently being observed in endemic areas [34]. In addition, regular clinical, radiological and parasitological monitoring after treatment is essential. Post-treatment monitoring involves checks at two, six months and one year. Resumption of treatment is recommended if the parasitological tests remain positive after three months. It should be noted, however, that none of our patients underwent parasitological checks.

Based on the results of this study, it is crucial not to limit screening for intestinal and urinary parasitosis to ENRPT. It should be extended to all people from regions endemic for emerging and re-emerging parasitoses who reside in Tunisia. Parasitological examinations of stools and urine should be systematically required, for example, during recruitment examinations for professionals on assignment in Tunisia. In addition, it would be beneficial to conduct multicentre studies involving all the laboratories that take samples of parasites. parasitological tests on ERNPT, in order to control the risk of reintroduction and spread of these parasites, by reviewing and adopting the best control measures.

CONCLUSIONS

Bilharziasis, also known as schistosomiasis, is an endemic tropical parasitic disease that is often neglected. They pose a major public health problem in the countries where they are most widespread, due to their high morbidity and mortality rates. In Tunisia, the last case of indigenous transmission was recorded in 1984, thanks to the implementation of a national programme to eradicate schistosomiasis. However, we are currently witnessing the emergence of a new epidemiological profile for bilharziasis: imported cases. As part of the surveillance and screening of emerging and re-emerging digestive and urinary parasitoses, ENRPTs must undergo a parasitological examination of their stools and urine before they can enrol in Tunis universities. The aim of this study was to analyse the epidemiological, clinical and parasitological characteristics of cases of bilharziasis diagnosed in ENRPTs. To this end, a descriptive cross-sectional study was conducted at the Parasitology-Mycology Laboratory of the Charles Nicolle Hospital over a period of 15 academic years, from 2008-2009 to 2022-2023. The study covered 6051 ENRPT enrolled in various public and private higher education establishments in the Tunis region. Each student underwent an interview and parasitological examinations of urine (based on direct microscopic observation) and stools (including a direct examination of the fresh state and a stool concentration technique: simplified Ritchie). During the study period, 91 cases of parasites were recorded, representing a frequency of 1.5%. Among the students affected, intestinal schistosomiasis was found in 83% of cases (N=76). A Urogenital schistosomiasis was diagnosed in 14 ENRPTs, with a combination of the two clinical forms in only one student. The trend in schistosomiasis cases over the years has shown great variability, with the highest number of cases recorded in the 2017-2018 academic year (19 cases), while no cases were diagnosed in the 2008-2009, 2010-2011 and 2022-2023 academic years. The study population had an average age of 24 years, with a clear male predominance (77%). All the parasites were from sub-Saharan Africa. Clinically, most of the students were asymptomatic.For cases of intestinal schistosomiasis, intestinal polyparasitism was observed in 47 ERNPT (62%), with one case having both clinical forms. Among those parasitized by S. haematobium, 8 students were carriers of other digestive parasites.The emergence of new outbreaks of urogenital bilharziasis remains possible in Tunisia as long as the reservoir of the disease exists in the world and the intermediate host (the bulin mollusc) is present in Tunisia. Consequently, it is necessary to maintain systematic screening for these conditions and to treat infected students effectively. On the other hand, S. mansoni does not pose a threat to the country, as the intermediate host required to complete its life cycle is absent in our climate. However, students infected with this schistosome may harbour other digestive parasites, underlining the importance of monitoring and screening for ERNPT through regular parasitological examinations.It is crucial not to restrict screening for intestinal and urinary parasitosis to students who are not permanent residents of Tunisia. It should be extended to all people from regions endemic for emerging and re-emerging parasitoses who reside in Tunisia.

REFERENCES

1. Dridi K, Fakhfakh N, Belhadj S, Kaouech E, Kallel K, Chaker E. Intestinal parasitosis among non-permanent resident students in tunisia: a review of 23 years of monitoring in the department of Parasitology-mycology at the Rabta hospital of Tunis. Tunis Med. 2015;93(7):436-9.

2. Siala E, Aoun K, Zallagua N, Maatoug R, Bouratbine A. Value of screening for intestinal and urinary parasites in non-resident permanent students in Tunisia. Arch Inst Pasteur Tunis. 2003;80(1-4):29-33.

3. Lingscheid T, Kurth F, Clerinx J, Marocco S, Trevino B, Schunk M, et al. Schistosomiasis in European Travelers and Migrants: Analysis of 14 Years TropNet Surveillance Data. Am J Trop Med Hyg. 2017;97(2):567-74.

4. Marchese V, Beltrame A, Angheben A, Monteiro GB, Giorli G, Perandin F, et al. Schistosomiasis in immigrants, refugees and travellers in an Italian referral centre for tropical diseases. Infect Dis Poverty. 2018;7(1):55.

5. Tilli M, Gobbi F, Rinaldi F, Testa J, Caligaris S, Magro P, et al. The diagnosis and treatment of urogenital schistosomiasis in Italy in a

retrospective cohort of immigrants from Sub-Saharan Africa. Infection. 2019;47(3):447-59.

6. Aula OP, McManus DP, Jones MK, Gordon CA. Schistosomiasis with a Focus on Africa. Trop Med Infect Dis. 2021;6(3):109.

7. Chaker E, Latiri Z, Gargouri S, et al. Les parasitoses chez les étudiants non-résidents en Tunisie: Intérêt des examens systématiques. Maghreb Med. 1991e éd. :36-40.

8. Bouratbine A, Aoun K, Siala E, Chahed MK, Hassine LB, Meherzi A. Pour une meilleure estimation de la prévalence du parasitisme intestinal dans la région de Tunis. Bull Soc Pathol Exot. 2000;93(5):353.

9. Comelli A, Genovese C, Gobbi F, Brindicci G, Capone S, Corpolongo A, et al. Schistosomiasis in non-endemic areas: Italian consensus recommendations for screening, diagnosis and management by the Italian Society of Tropical Medicine and Global Health (SIMET), endorsed by the Committee for the Study of Parasitology of the Italian Association of Clinical Microbiologists (CoSP-AMCLI), the Italian Society of Parasitology (SoIPa), the Italian Society of Gastroenterology and Digestive Endoscopy (SIGE), the Italian Society of Gynaecology and Obstetrics (SIGO), the Italian Society of Colposcopy and Cervico-Vaginal Pathology (SICPCV), the Italian

Society of General Medicine and Primary Care (SIMG), the Italian Society of Infectious and Tropical Diseases (SIMIT), the Italian Society of Pediatrics (SIP), the Italian Society of Paediatric Infectious Diseases (SITIP), the Italian Society of Urology (SIU). Infection. 2023;51(5):1249-71.

10. Norman FF, Monge-Maillo B, Martínez-Pérez Á, Perez-Molina JA, López-Vélez R. Parasitic infections in travelers and immigrants: part II helminths and ectoparasites. Future Microbiol. 2015;10(1):87-99.

11. Hawkins KR, Cantera JL, Storey HL, Leader BT, de Los Santos T. Diagnostic Tests to Support Late-Stage Control Programs for Schistosomiasis and Soil-Transmitted Helminthiases. PLoS Negl Trop Dis. 2016;10(12):e0004985.

12. Isaiah PM, Sólveig Palmeirim M, Steinmann P. Epidemiology of pediatric schistosomiasis in hard-to-reach areas and populations: a scoping review. Infect Dis Poverty. 2023;12(1):37.

13. Dai SM, Guan Z, Zhang LJ, Lv S, Cao CL, Li SZ, et al. Imported Schistosomiasis, China, 2010-2018. Emerg Infect Dis. 2020;26(1):179-80.

14. Gryseels B. Schistosomiasis. Infect Dis Clin North Am. 2012;26(2):383-97.

15. Trabelsi S, Bouchakoua M, Aouinet A, Sellami A, Khaled S. Is there any change in the prevalence of intestinal and urinary parasitosis among "non-permanent resident" students in Tunisia?

16. Keiser J, N'Goran EK, Traoré M, Lohourignon KL, Singer BH, Lengeler C, et al. Polyparasitism with schistosoma mansoni, geohelminths, and intestinal protozoa in rural côte d'ivoire. J Parasitol. 2002;88(3):461-6.

17. Carmoi T. EMC 2010 hepatology.

18. Buonfrate D, Gobbi F, Marchese V, Postiglione C, Monteiro GB, Giorli G, et al. Extended screening for infectious diseases among newly arrived asylum seekers from Africa and Asia, Verona province, Italy, April 2014 to June 2015. Eurosurveillance. 2018;23(16):17.

19. Delcor NS, Maruri BT, Arandes AS, Guiu IC, Essadik HO, Soley ME, et al. Infectious Diseases in Sub-Saharan Immigrants to Spain. Am J Trop Med Hyg. 2016;94(4):750- 6.

20. ANOFEL. Medical parasitology and mycology. 2017.

21. Roure S, Valerio L, Pérez-Quílez O, Fernández-Rivas G, Martínez-Cuevas O, Alcántara-Román A, et al. Epidemiological, clinical, diagnostic and economic features of an immigrant population of chronic schistosomiasis sufferers with long-term residence in a

nonendemic country (North Metropolitan area of Barcelona, 2002-2016). PLoS One. 2017;12(9):e0185245.

22. Milesi M, Indovina C, Dino O, Di Bella F, Di Lorenzo F, Sanfilippo A, et al. Urinary schistosomiasis in migrant population: a case series from a single centre in southern Italy. Infection. 2019;47(3):395-8.

23. Geremia N, De Vito A, Lai V, Fiore V, Princic E, Rappelli P, et al. Human urogenital schistosomiasis in West and Sub-Saharan Africa migrants in Sardinia, Italy: A retrospective monocentric study. J Infect Dev Ctries. 2022;16(08):1359-63.

24. Anisuzzaman, Tsuji N. Schistosomiasis and hookworm infection in humans: Disease burden, pathobiology and anthelmintic vaccines. Parasitol Int. 2020:75:102051.

25. Barakat RMR. Epidemiology of Schistosomiasis in Egypt: Travel through Time: Review. J Adv Res. 2013;4(5):425-32.

26. Hotez PJ, Savioli L, Fenwick A. Neglected Tropical Diseases of the Middle East and North Africa: Review of Their Prevalence, Distribution, and Opportunities for Control. PLoS Negl Trop Dis. 2012;6(2):e1475.

27. Ben Rachid MS, Ben Ammar R, Redissi T, Ben Said M, Hellal H, Bach-Hamba D, et al. Geography of major parasitosis in Tunisia. Arch

Inst Pasteur Tunis. 1984;61(1):17-41.

28. Rey L, MT H, Bahri M, Nacef T, Fareh R. Schistosomiasis in Tunisia. Résultats après dix ans de lutte contre l'endemie. 1982 [cited 21 Oct 2023]; Available from: https://pascalfrancis.inist.fr/vibad/index.php?action=getRecordDetail&idt=PASCAL8 3X0092371

29. Hariz MB, Farhat L, Hlioui S, Chourou O, Essafi-Kallel K, Mahjoub A, et al. Urinary bilharziasis: 9 imported cases. La Tunisie Medicale 2007;85(2) 150-154.

30. AFP S and A with. Sciences et Avenir. 2014 [cited 21 Oct 2023]. Bilharziasis, a tropical disease its apparition in Corse. Available https://www.sciencesetavenir.fr/sante/la-bilharziose-une-maladie-tropicale-fait- sonapparition-en-corse_27377

31. Deniaud F, Vignier N, Raynal G, Boo N, Collignon A, Hennequin C. Schistosoma haematobium urinary tract complications in African migrants attending primary care facilities in Paris, France: A retrospective cohort study (2004-2018). Infectious Diseases Now. 2023;53(6):104715.

32. Carbonell C, Rodríguez-Alonso B, López-Bernús A, Almeida H, Galindo-Pérez I, Velasco-Tirado V, et al. Clinical Spectrum of Schistosomiasis: An Update. J Clin Med. 2021;10(23):5521.

33. Sy I, Balde Y, Ndao B, Barbier D, Georges P, Ndir O. Bilharziosis in eastern Senegal. Eur j water qual. 2011;42(1):1-5.

34. Meltzer E, Schwartz E. Schistosomiasis: Current Epidemiology and Management in Travelers. Curr Infect Dis Rep. 2013;15(3):211-5.

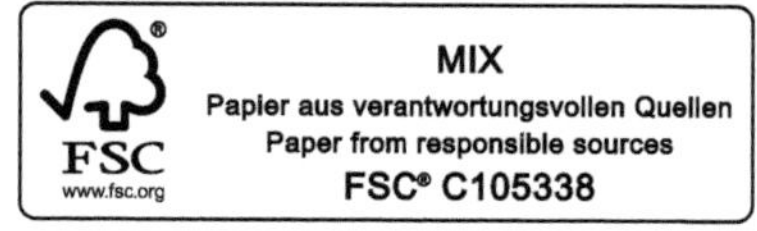

Printed by Books on Demand GmbH, Norderstedt / Germany